Keto Cookbook for Beginners (2021)

A Complete Guide to Effectively Lose Weight Fast with Delicious Low-Carb Recipes

Anne-Marie Wall

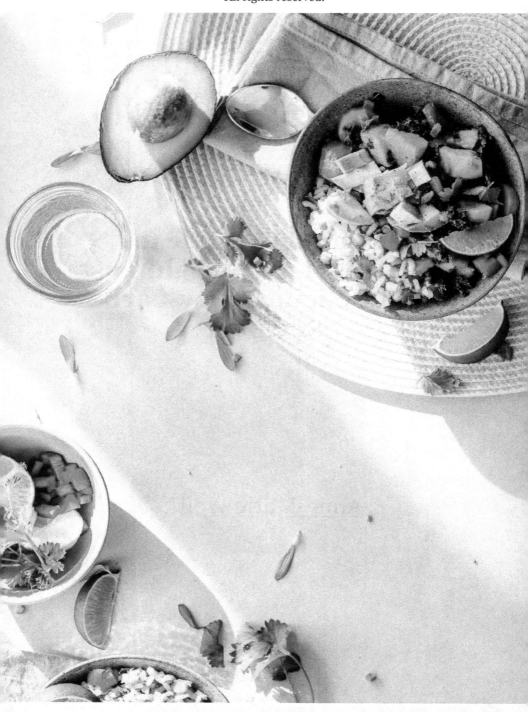

CONTENTS

Camembert & Chili Bacon Balls

Ingredients for 2 servings

- 1 cup bacon, finely chopped
- 5 oz camembert cheese, cubed
- 1 chili pepper, seeded and chopped
- ¼ tsp parsley flakes
- ½ tsp paprika

Instructions and Total Time: approx. 15 minutes

Fry the bacon in a pan over medium heat until crispy; about 5 minutes.

Let cool for a few minutes.

Place the camembert cheese, chili pepper, parsley, and paprika in a bowl
and mix to combine well.

Create balls from the mixture.

Set the cooled bacon in a plate.

Roll the balls around to coat all sides.

Nutrition Facts: Cal 456; Fat 39.5g; Net Carbs 3.6g; Protein 22.4g

Basil Spinach & Zucchini Lasagna

Ingredients for 4 servings

- 2 zucchinis, sliced
- Salt and black pepper to taste
- 2 cups feta cheese
- 2 cups mozzarella cheese, shredded
- 3 cups tomato sauce
- 1 cup spinach
- 1 tbsp basil, chopped

Instructions and Total Time: approx. 40 minutes

Preheat oven to 370 F.

Mix the feta, mozzarella cheese, salt, and black pepper to evenly combine and spread ¼ cup of the mixture at the bottom of a greased baking dish.

Layer 1/3 of the zucchini slices on top, spread 1 cup of tomato sauce over and scatter a 1/3 cup of spinach on top.

Repeat the layering process two more times to exhaust the **Ingredients** while making sure to layer with the last ¼ cup of cheese mixture finally.

Bake for 35 minutes until the cheese has a nice golden brown color.

Remove the dish, sit for 5 minutes and serve sprinkled with basil.

Nutrition Facts: Cal 411; Fat 43g; Net Carbs 3.2g; Protein 6.5g

Herbed Cheese Sticks with Yogurt Dip

Ingredients for 2 servings

- 8 oz mozzarella cheese, cut into sticks
- ¼ cup Parmesan cheese, grated
- 1 tbsp almond flour
- 1/3 tbsp flax meal
- 1/3 tsp cumin powder
- ½ tsp dried oregano
- 1/3 tsp dried rosemary
- 1 egg
- 1 tbsp olive oil

Yogurt dip

- 1/3 cup natural yogurt
- 1 garlic clove
- 1 tsp mint, chopped
- 1 tbsp parsley, chopped
- Sea salt to taste

Instructions and Total Time: approx. 40 minutes

In a bowl, mix the almond flour, flax meal, cumin powder, oregano, and rosemary.

In a separate bowl, whisk the egg with a fork.

Dip in each cheese stick into the egg, then roll in the dry mixture.

Set cheese sticks on a wax paper-lined baking sheet; freeze for 30 minutes.

In a skillet over medium heat warm oil and fry cheese sticks for 5 minutes until the coating is golden brown and crisp.

Set on paper towels to drain excess oil.

Mash the garlic and salt to taste into a pestle and add to the yogurt.

Stir in olive oil, parsley and mint.

Spread into a serving bowl and serve with the cheese sticks.

Nutrition Facts: Cal 354; Fat 15.9g; Net Carbs 3.7g; Protein 44.4g

Roasted Pumpkin with Almonds & Cheddar

Ingredients for 4 servings

- 2 tbsp olive oil
- 1 large pumpkin, peeled and sliced
- ½ cup almonds, ground
- ½ cup cheddar cheese, grated
- 2 tbsp thyme, chopped

Instructions and Total Time: approx. 45 minutes

Preheat the oven to 360 F.

Arrange pumpkin slices on a baking dish, drizzle with olive oil, and bake for 35 minutes.

Mix almonds and cheese, and when the pumpkin is ready, remove it from the oven, and sprinkle the cheese mixture all over.

Bake for 5 more minutes.

Sprinkle with thyme to serve.

Nutrition Facts: Cal 154; Fat 8.6g; Net Carbs 5.1g; Protein 4.5g

Avocado Crostini with Hazelnuts

Ingredients for 4 servings

- 2 avocados, chopped
- 4 tbsp olive oil
- 3 tbsp grated Parmesan
- 2 tbsp chopped hazelnuts
- 2 garlic cloves, halved
- ¼ tsp garlic powder
- ¼ tsp onion powder
- 1 tbsp chopped parsley
- 1 lemon, zested and juiced
- 1 loaf zero carb bread, sliced

Instructions and Total Time: approx. 25 minutes

In a bowl, place 2 tbsp olive oil, avocado, garlic and onion powders, salt, pepper, parsley, zest, and juice and mix with a fork until smooth; set aside.

Heat a grill pan.

Rub both sides of the bread slices with garlic and brush with remaining

olive oil.

Grill on both sides until crispy and golden.

Spread the avocado mixture onto the crostini.

Sprinkle with Parmesan cheese and hazelnuts.

Drizzle with some more olive oil and serve.

Nutrition Facts: Cal 331; Net Carbs 3.9g; Fat 29g; Protein 3.6g

Sesame Tofu Skewers

Ingredients for 4 servings

- 1 tbsp olive oil
- 1 (14 oz) firm tofu, cubed
- 1 zucchini, cut into wedges
- ¼ cup cherry tomatoes, halved
- 1 red onion, cut into wedges
- 2 tbsp tahini
- 1 tbsp soy sauce
- Sesame seeds for garnishing

Instructions and Total Time: approx. 15 min + marinating time

In a bowl, mix tahini and soy sauce.

Toss the tofu in the mixture.

Let rest for 30 minutes.

Thread tofu, zucchini, cherry tomatoes, and onion, alternately on skewers.

Brush with olive oil.

Heat a grill pan and cook tofu skewers until golden, 8 minutes.

Serve garnished with sesame seeds.

Nutrition Facts: Cal 271; Net Carbs 2.4g; Fat 17g; Protein 14g

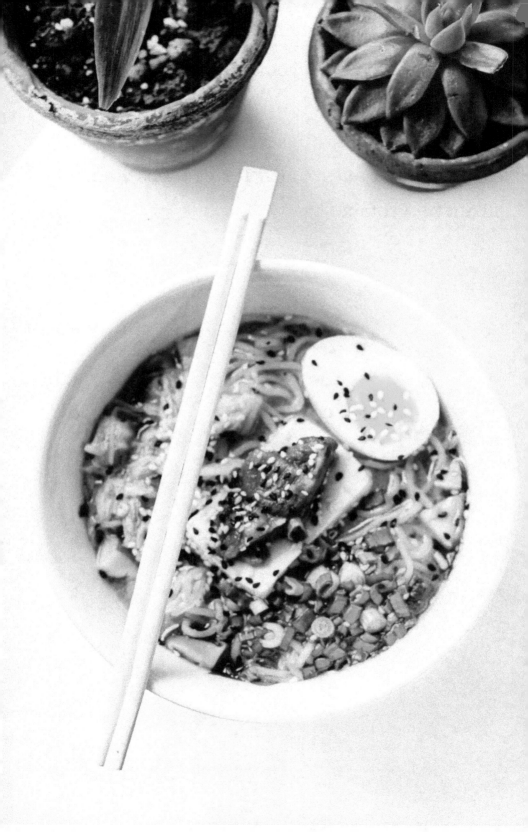

Parmigiano Cauliflower Cakes

Ingredients for 4 servings

- 2 cups cauliflower florets
- ½ cup grated Parmigiano cheese
- 1 cup olive oil
- 1 large egg, beaten
- 2 green onions, chopped
- 1 tbsp chopped parsley
- 2 tbsp chopped almonds
- 1 cup golden flaxseed meal
- Salt and black pepper to taste

Instructions and Total Time: approx. 25 minutes

Place cauliflower and 1 cup of water into a pot and bring to a boil until soft;

drain.

Transfer to a food processor.

Puree until smooth.

Pour into a bowl and mix in salt, pepper, egg, green onions, parsley,

cheese, and almonds.

Make 12 small cakes from the mixture and coat with the flaxseed meal.

Heat olive oil a deep pan and cook patties on both sides until golden, 6-8

minutes.

Serve warm.

Nutrition Facts: Cal 319; Net Carbs 5.5g; Fat 19g; Protein 14g

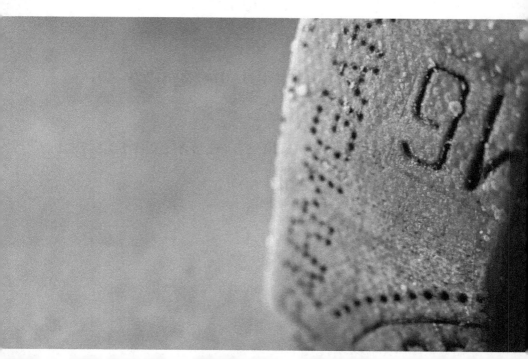

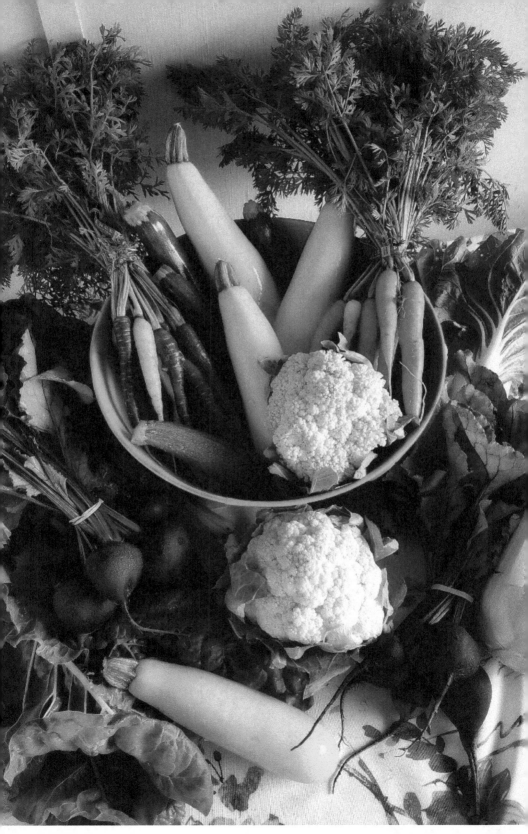

Raspberry & Goat Cheese Focaccia Bites

Ingredients for 6 servings

- 6 zero carb buns, cut into 4 squares each
- 1 cup mushrooms, sliced
- 1 cup fresh raspberries
- 2 cups erythritol
- 1 lemon, juiced
- 1 tbsp olive oil
- ½ tsp dried thyme
- 2 oz goat cheese, crumbled
- 1 green onion, chopped

Instructions and Total Time: approx. 25 minutes

Place raspberries into a saucepan, break into a puree using a potato

masher, and stir in erythritol and lemon juice.

Place the pot over low heat and cook with constant stirring until the sugar dissolves.

Turn the heat up to medium and let the mixture boil for 4 minutes, still with constant stirring to prevent the jam from burning; let cool.

Preheat oven to 350 F.

Arrange the buns on a baking tray and bake for 6 minutes.

Heat olive oil in a skillet and sauté mushrooms with thyme for 10 minutes.

Remove the bread squares from the oven, cut each square into halves horizontally, and top with mushrooms.

Scatter with goat cheese, green onion, and raspberry jam.

Cover with 6 pieces of focaccia and serve.

Nutrition Facts: Cal 171; Net Carbs 5.7g; Fat 9g; Protein 7g

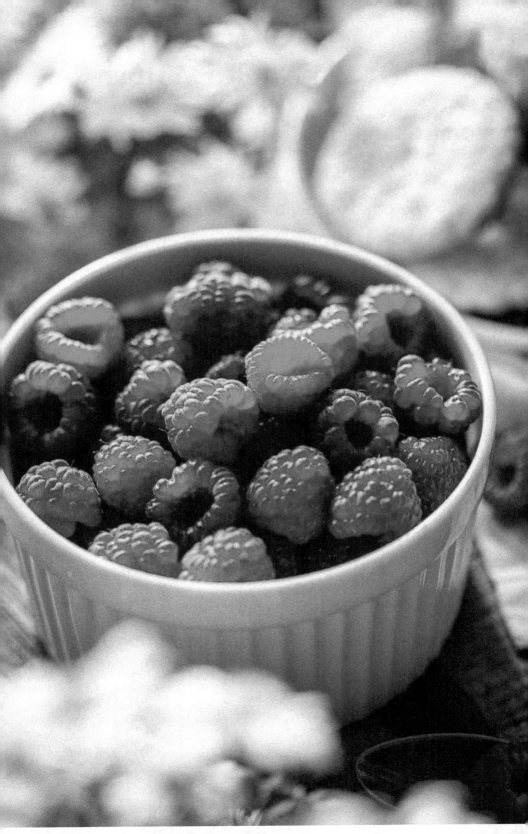

Green Nacho Wings

Ingredients for 4 servings

- 16 chicken wings, halved
- ½ cup butter, melted
- 1 lb grated Mexican cheese blend
- 1 cup golden flaxseed meal
- 2 tbsp chopped green chilies
- 1 cup chopped scallions
- 1 jalapeño pepper, sliced

Instructions and Total Time: approx. 45 minutes

Preheat oven to 360 F.

Brush the chicken with butter.

Spread the flaxseed meal on a wide plate and roll in each chicken wing.

Place on a baking sheet and bake for 30-35 minutes or until golden brown
and cooked within.

Sprinkle with the cheese blend, green chilies,
scallions, and jalapeño

pepper on top.

Serve immediately.

Nutrition Facts: Cal 802; Net Carbs 1.5g;

Fat 59g; Protein 51g

Eggplant & Bacon Gratin

Ingredients for 4 servings

- 3 large eggplants, sliced
- 6 bacon slices, chopped
- ½ cup shredded Parmesan
- ½ cup crumbled feta cheese
- 1 tbsp dried oregano
- ¾ cup heavy cream
- 2 tbsp chopped parsley
- Salt and black pepper to taste

Instructions and Total Time: approx. 50 minutes

Preheat oven to 380 F.

Put bacon in a skillet and fry over medium heat until brown and crispy, 6 minutes.

Transfer to a plate.

Arrange half of eggplants in a greased baking sheet and season with
oregano, parsley, salt, and pepper.
Scatter half of bacon and half of feta cheese on top and repeat the layering
process using the remaining **Ingredients**.
In a bowl, combine heavy cream with half of the Parmesan cheese, and
spread on top of the layered **Ingredients**.
Sprinkle with the remaining Parmesan.
Bake until the cream is bubbly and the gratin golden, 20 minutes.
Serve.

Nutrition Facts: Cal 429; Net Carbs 1.7g; Fat 30g; Protein 16g

Bacon Wrapped Halloumi

Ingredients for 4 servings

- 16 bacon strips
- ½ lb halloumi cheese, cubed
- ½ cup swerve brown sugar
- ½ cup mayonnaise
- ¼ cup hot sauce

Instructions and Total Time: approx. 30 minutes

Place the bacon in a skillet and cook over medium heat on both sides until crisp, 5 minutes; transfer to a plate.

Wrap each halloumi cheese with a bacon strip and secure with a toothpick each.

Place on a baking sheet.

In a bowl, combine swerve brown sugar, mayonnaise, and hot sauce.

Pour the mixture all over the bacon-halloumi pieces and bake in the oven at
350 F for 10 minutes.

Serve chilled.

Nutrition Facts: Cal 351; Net Carbs 4.6g; Fat 24.9g; Protein 13g

Mini Sausages with Sweet Mustard Sauce

Ingredients for 4 servings

- 2 lb mini smoked sausages
- 3 tbsp almond flour
- 2 tsp mustard powder
- ¼ cup lemon juice
- ¼ cup white wine vinegar
- 1 cup swerve brown sugar
- 1 tsp tamari sauce

Instructions and Total Time: approx. 15 minutes

In a pot, combine swerve brown sugar, almond flour, and mustard.

Gradually stir in lemon juice, vinegar, and tamari sauce.

Bring to a boil over medium heat while stirring until thickened, 2 minutes.

Mix in sausages until properly coated.

Cook them for 5 minutes.

Serve warm.

Nutrition Facts: Cal 751; Net Carbs 7.2g; Fat 44.8g; Protein 24g

Pancetta & Broccoli Roast

Ingredients for 4 servings

- 6 pancetta slices, chopped
- 1 lb broccoli rabe, halved
- 2 tbsp olive oil
- ¼ tsp red chili flakes

Instructions and Total Time: approx. 40 minutes

Preheat oven to 420 F.

Place broccoli rabe in a greased baking sheet and top with pancetta.

Drizzle with olive oil, season to taste, and sprinkle with chili flakes.

Roast for 30 minutes.

Serve warm and enjoy!

Nutrition Facts: Cal 130; Net Carbs 0.2g; Fat 10g; Protein 6.8g

Mushroom & Kale Pierogis

Ingredients for 4 servings

- 2 oz fresh kale
- 3 oz bella mushrooms, sliced
- ½ cup cream cheese
- 2 cups Parmesan, grated
- 7 tbsp butter
- 2 garlic cloves, minced
- 1 small red onion, chopped
- 3 eggs
- ½ cup almond flour
- 4 tbsp coconut flour
- 1 tsp baking powder
- Salt and black pepper to taste

Instructions and Total Time: approx. 45 minutes

Melt 2 tbsp of butter in a skillet and sauté garlic, red onion, mushrooms, and kale for 5 minutes.

Season with salt and pepper and reduce the heat to low.

Stir in cream cheese and ½ cup of Parmesan cheese; simmer for 1 minute.

Set aside to cool.

In a bowl, combine almond and coconut flours, salt, and baking powder.

Put a pan over low heat and melt the remaining Parmesan cheese and butter.

Turn the heat off.

Pour the eggs in the cream mixture, continue stirring, while adding the flour mixture until a firm dough forms.

Mold the dough into balls, place on a chopping board, and use a rolling pin to flatten each into ½ inch thin round piece.

Spread a generous amount of stuffing on one-half of each dough, fold over the filling, and seal the dough with fingers. Brush with oil and bake for 20 minutes at 380 F.

Nutrition Facts: Cal 538; Net Carbs 6g; Fat 51g; Protein 18g

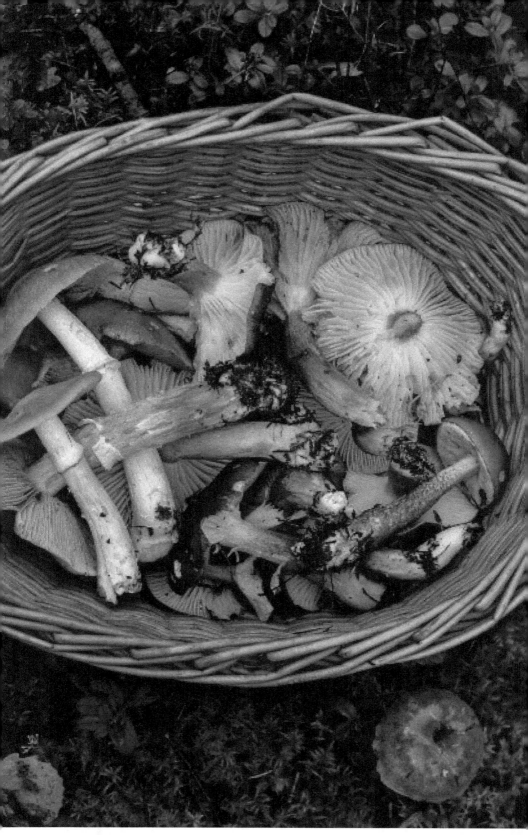

Chicken Ranch Pizza with Bacon & Basil

Ingredients for 4 servings

- 1 tbsp butter
- 2 chicken breasts
- 3 cups shredded mozzarella
- 3 tbsp cream cheese, softened
- ¾ cup almond flour
- 2 tbsp almond meal
- ¼ cup half and half
- 1 tbsp dry Ranch seasoning
- 3 bacon slices, chopped
- 6 fresh basil leaves

Instructions and Total Time: approx. 45 minutes

Preheat oven to 390 F.

Line a pizza pan with parchment paper.

Microwave 2 cups of mozzarella cheese and 2 tbsp of the cream cheese
for 30 seconds.

Mix in almond flour and almond meal.

Spread the "dough" on the pan and bake for 15 minutes.

In a bowl, mix butter, remaining cream cheese, half and half, and ranch
mix; set aside.

Heat a grill pan and cook the bacon for 5 minutes; set aside.

Grill the chicken in the pan on both sides for 10 minutes.

Remove to a plate, allow cooling and cut into thin slices.

Spread the ranch sauce on the pizza crust, followed by the chicken and
bacon, and then, the remaining mozzarella cheese and basil.

Bake for 5 minutes.

Serve sliced.

Nutrition Facts: Cal 531; Net Carbs 4g; Fats 32g; Protein 62g

Pizza Bianca with Mushrooms

Ingredients for 2 servings

- 2 tbsp olive oil
- 4 eggs
- 2 tbsp water
- 1 jalapeño pepper, diced
- ¼ cup mozzarella, shredded
- 2 chives, chopped
- 2 cups egg Alfredo sauce
- ½ tsp oregano
- ½ cup mushrooms, sliced

Instructions and Total Time: approx. 17 minutes

Preheat oven to 360 F.

In a bowl, whisk eggs, water, and oregano.

Heat the olive oil in a large skillet.

Pour in the egg mixture and cook until set, flipping once.

Remove and spread the alfredo sauce and jalapeño pepper all over.

Top with mozzarella cheese, mushrooms and chives.

Bake for 5-10 minutes until the cheese melts.

Nutrition Facts: Cal 312; Fat 24g; Net Carbs 2.4g; Protein 17g

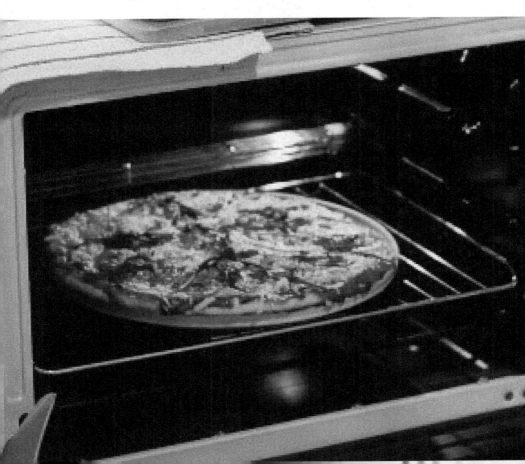

Kale & Cheese Stuffed Zucchini

Ingredients for 2 servings

- 1 zucchini, halved
- 4 tbsp butter
- 2 garlic cloves, minced
- 1 ½ oz baby kale
- Salt and black pepper to taste
- 2 tbsp unsweetened tomato sauce
- 1 cup mozzarella cheese, shredded
- Olive oil for drizzling

Instructions and Total Time: approx. 40 minutes

Preheat oven to 375 F.

Scoop out the pulp of the zucchini with a spoon into a plate; keep the flesh.

Grease a baking sheet with cooking spray and place the zucchini halves on top.

Put the butter in a skillet and melt over medium heat.

Add and sauté the garlic until fragrant and slightly browned, about 4 minutes.

Add the kale and the zucchini pulp.

Cook until the kale wilts; season with salt and black pepper.

Spoon the tomato sauce into the zucchini halves and spread to coat the bottom evenly.

Spoon the kale mixture into the zucchinis and sprinkle with the mozzarella cheese.

Bake in the oven for 20 to 25 minutes or until the cheese has a beautiful golden color.

Plate the zucchinis when ready, drizzle with olive oil, and season with salt and black pepper.

Nutrition Facts: Cal 345; Fat 25g; Net Carbs 6.9g; Protein 2g

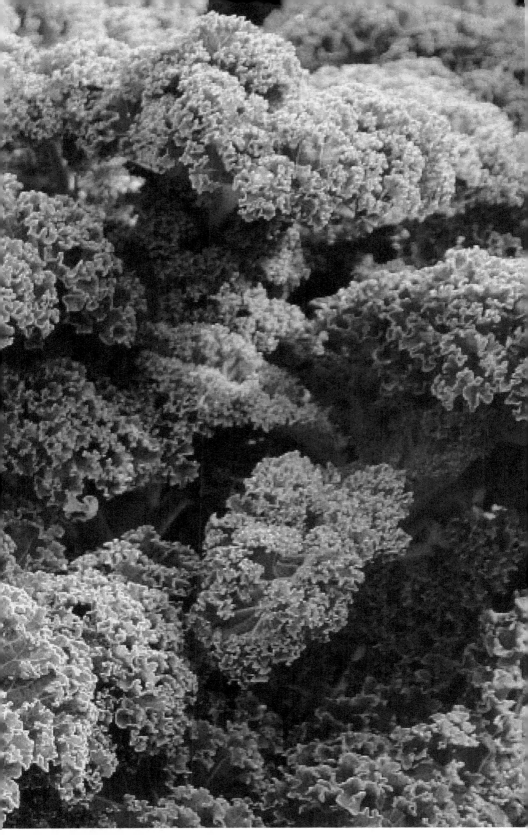

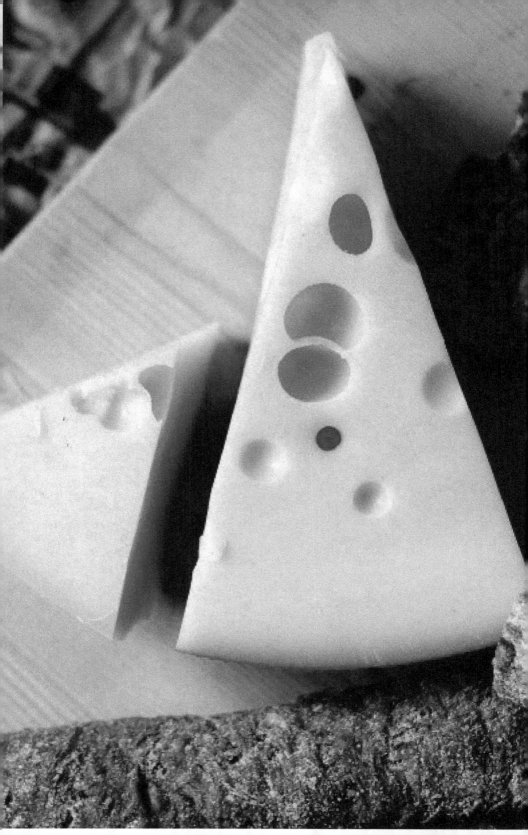

Italian Turnip Bites

Ingredients for 4 servings

- ¼ cup grated mozzarella
- 1 lb turnips, sliced into rounds
- ¼ cup marinara sauce
- ½ cup olive oil
- 2 garlic cloves, minced
- 1 tbsp chopped fresh parsley
- 2 tbsp chopped fresh oregano
- 3 tbsp dried Italian seasoning

Instructions and Total Time: approx. 1 hour

Preheat oven to 400 F.

Place turnip slices into a bowl and toss with olive oil.

Add in garlic, oregano, and Italian seasoning and mix well.

Arrange on a greased baking sheet and roast for 25 minutes, flipping
halfway.

Remove and brush with the marinara sauce.

Sprinkle with mozzarella cheese and bake in the oven until the cheese is
melted and golden, 15 minutes.

Garnish with parsley and serve warm.

Nutrition Facts: Cal 331; Net Carbs 3.8g; Fat 28g; Protein 5g

Healthy Turnip Fries

Ingredients for 4 servings

- 3 tbsp olive oil
- 4 large parsnips, sliced
- 3 tbsp ground pork rinds
- ¼ tsp red chili flakes

Instructions and Total Time: approx. 50 minutes

Preheat oven to 420 F.

Pour parsnips into a bowl and add in the pork rinds.

Toss and place the parsnips a baking sheet.

Drizzle with olive oil and sprinkle with chili flakes.

Bake until crispy, 40-45 minutes, tossing halfway.

Serve.

Nutrition Facts: Cal 259; Net Carbs 22.6g; Fat 10.8g; Protein 2.9g

Minute Steak & Radish Stir-Fry

Ingredients for 4 servings

- 10 oz minute steak
- 3 tbsp butter
- 1½ lb radishes, quartered
- 1 garlic clove, minced
- 2 tbsp freshly chopped thyme

Instructions and Total Time: approx. 30 minutes

Cut the meat into small pieces.

Melt butter in a skillet over medium heat, season the meat with salt and

pepper, and brown it until brown on all sides, 12 minutes; transfer to a

plate.

Add and sauté radishes, garlic, and thyme until the radishes are cooked, 10 minutes.

Plate and serve warm.

Nutrition Facts: Cal 249; Net Carbs 0.4g;
Fat 16g; Protein 21g

Creamy Celeriac & Bacon Bake

Ingredients for 4 servings

- 3 tbsp butter
- 6 bacon slices, chopped
- 3 garlic cloves, minced
- 3 tbsp almond flour
- 2 cups coconut cream
- 1 cup chicken broth
- 1 lb celeriac, peeled and sliced
- 2 cups shredded cheddar
- ¼ cup chopped scallions

- Salt and black pepper to taste

Instructions and Total Time: approx. 50 minutes

Preheat oven to 380 F.

Add bacon to a skillet and fry over medium heat until brown and crispy.

Spoon onto a plate.

Melt butter in the same skillet and sauté garlic for 1 minute.

Mix in almond flour and cook for another minute.

Whisk in coconut cream, chicken broth, salt, and pepper.

Simmer for 5 minutes.

Spread a layer of the sauce in a greased casserole dish and arrange layer celeriac on top.

Cover with more sauce, top with some bacon and cheddar cheese, and scatter scallions on top.

Repeat the layering process until the **Ingredients** are exhausted.

Bake for 35 minutes.

Let rest for a few minutes and serve.

Nutrition Facts: Cal 979; Net Carbs 20g; Fat 79g; Protein 30g

Gruyere & Chicken Ham Stuffed Peppers

Ingredients for 4 servings

- 12 mini green bell peppers, halved
- 4 slices chicken ham, chopped
- 2 tbsp melted butter
- 1 cup shredded Gruyere
- 1 tbsp chopped parsley
- 8 oz cream cheese
- ½ tbsp hot sauce

Instructions and Total Time: approx. 30 minutes

Preheat oven to 380 F.

Place peppers in a greased baking dish and set aside.

In a bowl, combine chicken ham, parsley, cream cheese, hot sauce, and butter.

Spoon the mixture into the peppers and sprinkle Gruyere cheese on top.

Bake until the cheese melts, about 20 minutes.

Serve.

Nutrition Facts: Cal 398; Net Carbs 4g; Fat 32g; Protein 20g

Serrano Ham & Asparagus Bake

Ingredients for 4 servings

- 1 cup grated Pecorino cheese
- 1 cup grated mozzarella
- 2 lb asparagus, stalks trimmed
- 4 slices Serrano ham, chopped
- ¾ cup coconut cream
- 3 garlic cloves, minced
- 1 cup crushed pork rinds
- ½ tsp sweet paprika

Instructions and Total Time: approx. 40 minutes

Preheat oven to 380 F.

Arrange asparagus on a greased baking dish and pour coconut cream on top.

Scatter the garlic, serrano ham, and pork rinds on top and sprinkle with Pecorino cheese, mozzarella cheese, and paprika.

Bake until the cheese melts and is golden and asparagus tender, 30 minutes.

Serve warm.

Nutrition Facts: Cal 359; Net Carbs 15g; Fat 19g; Protein 29g

Gruyere & Bacon Bites

Ingredients for 4 servings

- 6 oz cream cheese
- 6 oz shredded Gruyere cheese
- 7 bacon slices
- 2 tbsp butter, softened
- ½ tsp red chili flakes

Instructions and Total Time: approx. 30 minutes

Place the bacon in a skillet and fry over medium heat until crispy, 5
minutes.

Transfer to a plate to cool and crumble it.

Pour the bacon grease into a bowl and mix in cream cheese, Gruyere
cheese, butter, and red chili flakes.

Refrigerate to set for 15 minutes.

Remove and mold into walnut-sized balls.

Roll in the crumbled bacon.

Plate and serve.

Nutrition Facts: Cal 541; Net Carbs 0.5g; Fat 49g; Protein 22g

Cheddar & Salami Skewers

Ingredients for 4 servings

- 4 oz hard salami, cubed
- 12 oz cheddar cheese, cubed
- ¼ cup pitted Kalamata olives
- ¼ cup olive oil
- 1 tbsp plain vinegar
- 2 garlic cloves, minced
- 1 tsp dried Italian herb blend
- 1 tsp chopped parsley

Instructions and Total Time: approx. 10 min + chilling time

In a bowl, mix olive oil, vinegar, garlic, and herb blend.

Add in salami, olives, and cheddar cheese.
Mix until well coated.

Cover the bowl with plastic wrap and marinate in the refrigerator for 4 hours.

Remove, drain the marinade and thread one salami cube, one olive, and one cheese cube on a skewer.

Repeat making more skewers with the remaining **Ingredients**.

Garnish with parsley and serve.

Nutrition Facts: Cal 591; Net Carbs 1.8g; Fat 49g; Protein 27g

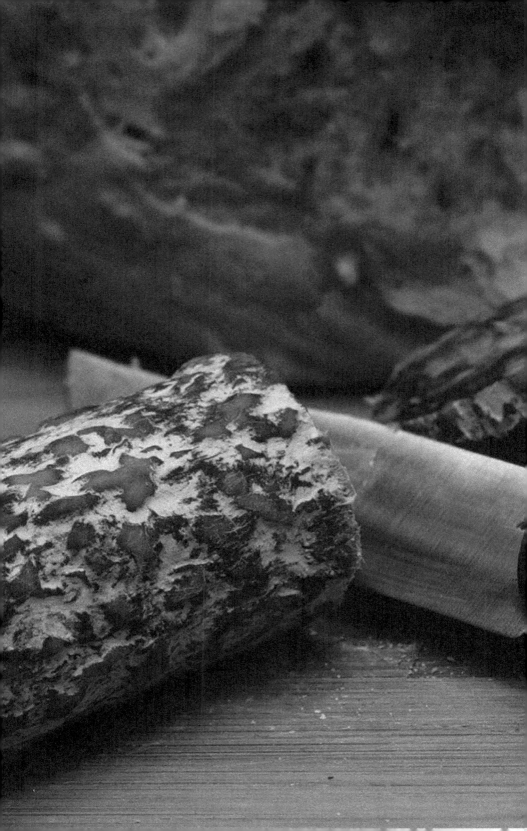

Parsley Cauliflower & Bacon Stir-Fry

Ingredients for 4 servings

- 10 oz bacon, chopped
- 1 head cauliflower, cut into florets
- 1 garlic clove, minced
- 2 tbsp parsley, finely chopped
- Salt and black pepper to taste

Instructions and Total Time: approx. 15 minutes

Throw the cauliflower in salted boiling water over medium heat and cook for

5 minutes or until soft; drain and set aside.

In a skillet, fry bacon until brown and crispy, 5 minutes.

Add cauliflower and garlic and sauté until the cauliflower browns slightly.

Season with salt and pepper.

Garnish with parsley and serve.

Nutrition Facts: Cal 239; Net Carbs 3.9g; Fat 21g; Protein 8.9g

Cheesy Green Bean & Bacon Roast

Ingredients for 4 servings

- 1 egg, beaten
- 5 tbsp grated mozzarella
- 2 tbsp olive oil
- 1 tsp onion powder
- 15 oz fresh green beans
- 4 bacon slices, chopped

Instructions and Total Time: approx. 30 minutes

Preheat oven to 360 F.

Line a baking sheet with parchment paper.

In a bowl, mix olive oil, onion and garlic powders, and egg.

Add in green beans and mozzarella cheese and toss to coat.

Pour the mixture onto the baking sheet and bake until the green beans

brown slightly and cheese melts, 20 minutes.

Fry bacon in a skillet until crispy and brown.

Remove green beans and divide between serving plates.

Top with bacon and serve.

Nutrition Facts: Cal 210; Net Carbs 2.6g; Fat 19g; Protein 5.9g

Artichoke & Bacon Gratin with Cauli Rice

Ingredients for 4 servings

- 1 cup canned artichoke hearts
- 6 bacon slices, chopped
- 2 cups cauliflower rice
- 3 cups baby spinach, chopped
- 1 garlic clove, minced
- 1 tbsp olive oil
- Salt and black pepper to taste
- ¼ cup sour cream
- 8 oz cream cheese, softened
- ¼ cup grated Parmesan
- 1 ½ cups grated mozzarella

Instructions and Total Time: approx. 30 minutes

Draine and chop the artichokes; set aside.

Preheat oven to 360 F.

Cook bacon in a skillet over medium heat until brown and crispy, 5 minutes.

Spoon onto a plate.

In a bowl, mix cauli rice, artichokes, spinach, garlic, olive oil, salt, pepper,

sour cream, cream cheese, bacon, and half of Parmesan cheese.

Spread the mixture onto a baking dish and top with the remaining

Parmesan and mozzarella cheeses.

Bake for 15 minutes.

Serve.

Nutrition Facts: Cal 498; Net Carbs 5.3g; Fat 41g; Protein 28g

Pancetta-Wrapped Strawberries

Ingredients for 4 servings

- 12 fresh strawberries
- 12 thin pancetta slices
- 1 cup mascarpone cheese
- 2 tbsp swerve confectioner's sugar
- 1/8 tsp white pepper

Instructions and Total Time: approx. 30 minutes

In a bowl, combine mascarpone, swerve confectioner's sugar, and white pepper.

Coat strawberries in the mixture, wrap each strawberry in a pancetta slice,

and place on an ungreased baking sheet.

Bake in the oven at 425 F for 15-20 minutes until pancetta browns.

Serve warm.

Nutrition Facts: Cal 169; Net Carbs 1.2g; Fat 10.9g; Protein 12g

Oregano Parsnip Mash with Ham

Ingredients for 4 servings

- 3 tbsp olive oil
- 4 tbsp butter
- 1 lb parsnips, diced
- 2 tsp garlic powder
- ¾ cup almond milk
- 4 tbsp heavy cream
- 6 slices deli ham, chopped
- 2 tsp freshly chopped oregano

Instructions and Total Time: approx. 45 minutes

Preheat oven to 380 F.

Spread parsnips on a baking sheet and drizzle with 2 tbsp olive oil.

Cover tightly with aluminum foil and bake until the parsnips are tender, 40 minutes.

Remove from the oven, take off the foil, and transfer to a bowl.

Add in garlic powder, almond milk, heavy cream, and butter.

With an immersion blender, puree the **Ingredients** until smooth.

Fold in the ham and sprinkle with oregano. Serve.

Nutrition Facts: Cal 480; Net Carbs 20g; Fat 29g; Protein 9.8g

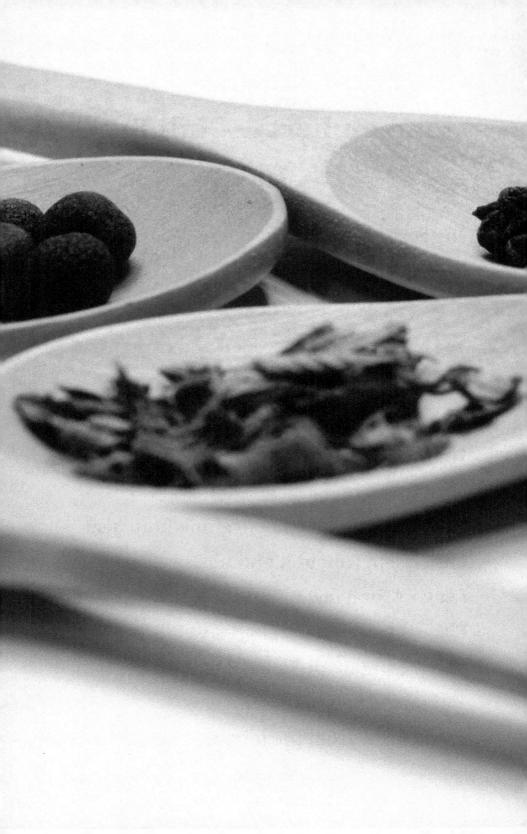

Camembert & Chili Bacon Balls

Ingredients for 2 servings

- 1 cup bacon, finely chopped
- 5 oz camembert cheese, cubed
- 1 chili pepper, seeded and chopped
- ¼ tsp parsley flakes
- ½ tsp paprika

Instructions and Total Time: approx. 15 minutes

Fry the bacon in a pan over medium heat until crispy; about 5 minutes.

Let cool for a few minutes.

Place the camembert cheese, chili pepper, parsley, and paprika in a bowl
and mix to combine well.

Create balls from the mixture.

Set the cooled bacon in a plate.

Roll the balls around to coat all sides.

Nutrition Facts: Cal 456; Fat 39.5g; Net Carbs 3.6g; Protein 22.4g

Basil Spinach & Zucchini Lasagna

Ingredients for 4 servings

- 2 zucchinis, sliced
- Salt and black pepper to taste
- 2 cups feta cheese
- 2 cups mozzarella cheese, shredded
- 3 cups tomato sauce
- 1 cup spinach
- 1 tbsp basil, chopped

Instructions and Total Time: approx. 40 minutes

Preheat oven to 370 F.

Mix the feta, mozzarella cheese, salt, and black pepper to evenly combine

and spread ¼ cup of the mixture at the bottom of a greased baking dish.

Layer 1/3 of the zucchini slices on top, spread 1 cup of tomato sauce over

and scatter a 1/3 cup of spinach on top.

Repeat the layering process two more times to exhaust the **Ingredients**

while making sure to layer with the last ¼ cup of cheese mixture finally.

Bake for 35 minutes until the cheese has a nice golden brown color.

Remove the dish, sit for 5 minutes and serve sprinkled with basil.

Nutrition Facts: Cal 411; Fat 43g; Net Carbs 3.2g; Protein 6.5g

Herbed Cheese Sticks with Yogurt Dip

Ingredients for 2 servings

- 8 oz mozzarella cheese, cut into sticks
- ¼ cup Parmesan cheese, grated
- 1 tbsp almond flour
- 1/3 tbsp flax meal
- 1/3 tsp cumin powder
- ½ tsp dried oregano
- 1/3 tsp dried rosemary
- 1 egg
- 1 tbsp olive oil

Yogurt dip

- 1/3 cup natural yogurt
- 1 garlic clove
- 1 tsp mint, chopped
- 1 tbsp parsley, chopped
- Sea salt to taste

Instructions and Total Time: approx. 40 minutes

In a bowl, mix the almond flour, flax meal, cumin powder, oregano, and rosemary.

In a separate bowl, whisk the egg with a fork.

Dip in each cheese stick into the egg, then roll in the dry mixture.

Set cheese sticks on a wax paper-lined baking sheet; freeze for 30 minutes.

In a skillet over medium heat warm oil and fry cheese sticks for 5 minutes until the coating is golden brown and crisp.

Set on paper towels to drain excess oil.

Mash the garlic and salt to taste into a pestle and add to the yogurt.

Stir in olive oil, parsley and mint.

Spread into a serving bowl and serve with the cheese sticks.

Nutrition Facts: Cal 354; Fat 15.9g; Net Carbs 3.7g; Protein 44.4g

Roasted Pumpkin with Almonds & Cheddar

Ingredients for 4 servings

- 2 tbsp olive oil
- 1 large pumpkin, peeled and sliced
- ½ cup almonds, ground
- ½ cup cheddar cheese, grated
- 2 tbsp thyme, chopped

Instructions and Total Time: approx. 45 minutes

Preheat the oven to 360 F.

Arrange pumpkin slices on a baking dish, drizzle with olive oil, and bake for 35 minutes.

Mix almonds and cheese, and when the pumpkin is ready, remove it from the oven, and sprinkle the cheese mixture all over.

Bake for 5 more minutes.

Sprinkle with thyme to serve.

Nutrition Facts: Cal 154; Fat 8.6g; Net Carbs 5.1g; Protein 4.5g

Avocado Crostini with Hazelnuts

Ingredients for 4 servings

- 2 avocados, chopped
- 4 tbsp olive oil
- 3 tbsp grated Parmesan
- 2 tbsp chopped hazelnuts
- 2 garlic cloves, halved
- ¼ tsp garlic powder
- ¼ tsp onion powder
- 1 tbsp chopped parsley
- 1 lemon, zested and juiced
- 1 loaf zero carb bread, sliced

Instructions and Total Time: approx. 25 minutes

In a bowl, place 2 tbsp olive oil, avocado, garlic and onion powders, salt, pepper, parsley, zest, and juice and mix with a fork until smooth; set aside.

Heat a grill pan.

Rub both sides of the bread slices with garlic and brush with remaining

olive oil.

Grill on both sides until crispy and golden.

Spread the avocado mixture onto the crostini.

Sprinkle with Parmesan cheese and hazelnuts.

Drizzle with some more olive oil and serve.

Nutrition Facts: Cal 331; Net Carbs 3.9g; Fat 29g; Protein 3.6g

Sesame Tofu Skewers

Ingredients for 4 servings

- 1 tbsp olive oil
- 1 (14 oz) firm tofu, cubed
- 1 zucchini, cut into wedges
- ¼ cup cherry tomatoes, halved
- 1 red onion, cut into wedges
- 2 tbsp tahini
- 1 tbsp soy sauce
- Sesame seeds for garnishing

Instructions and Total Time: approx. 15 min + marinating time

In a bowl, mix tahini and soy sauce.

Toss the tofu in the mixture.

Let rest for 30 minutes.

Thread tofu, zucchini, cherry tomatoes, and onion, alternately on skewers.

Brush with olive oil.

Heat a grill pan and cook tofu skewers until golden, 8 minutes.

Serve garnished with sesame seeds.

Nutrition Facts: Cal 271; Net Carbs 2.4g; Fat 17g; Protein 14g

Parmigiano Cauliflower Cakes

Ingredients for 4 servings

- 2 cups cauliflower florets
- ½ cup grated Parmigiano cheese
- 1 cup olive oil
- 1 large egg, beaten
- 2 green onions, chopped
- 1 tbsp chopped parsley
- 2 tbsp chopped almonds
- 1 cup golden flaxseed meal
- Salt and black pepper to taste

Instructions and Total Time: approx. 25 minutes

Place cauliflower and 1 cup of water into a pot and bring to a boil until soft;

drain.

Transfer to a food processor.

Puree until smooth.

Pour into a bowl and mix in salt, pepper, egg, green onions, parsley,

cheese, and almonds.

Make 12 small cakes from the mixture and coat with the flaxseed meal.

Heat olive oil a deep pan and cook patties on both sides until golden, 6-8

minutes.

Serve warm.

Nutrition Facts: Cal 319; Net Carbs 5.5g; Fat 19g; Protein 14g

Raspberry & Goat Cheese Focaccia Bites

Ingredients for 6 servings

- 6 zero carb buns, cut into 4 squares each
- 1 cup mushrooms, sliced
- 1 cup fresh raspberries
- 2 cups erythritol
- 1 lemon, juiced
- 1 tbsp olive oil
- ½ tsp dried thyme
- 2 oz goat cheese, crumbled
- 1 green onion, chopped

Instructions and Total Time: approx. 25 minutes

Place raspberries into a saucepan, break into a puree using a potato

masher, and stir in erythritol and lemon juice.

Place the pot over low heat and cook with constant stirring until the sugar dissolves.

Turn the heat up to medium and let the mixture boil for 4 minutes, still with constant stirring to prevent the jam from burning; let cool.

Preheat oven to 350 F.

Arrange the buns on a baking tray and bake for 6 minutes.

Heat olive oil in a skillet and sauté mushrooms with thyme for 10 minutes.

Remove the bread squares from the oven, cut each square into halves horizontally, and top with mushrooms.

Scatter with goat cheese, green onion, and raspberry jam.

Cover with 6 pieces of focaccia and serve.

Nutrition Facts: Cal 171; Net Carbs 5.7g; Fat 9g; Protein 7g

Green Nacho Wings

Ingredients for 4 servings

- 16 chicken wings, halved
- ½ cup butter, melted
- 1 lb grated Mexican cheese blend
- 1 cup golden flaxseed meal
- 2 tbsp chopped green chilies
- 1 cup chopped scallions
- 1 jalapeño pepper, sliced

Instructions and Total Time: approx. 45 minutes

Preheat oven to 360 F.

Brush the chicken with butter.

Spread the flaxseed meal on a wide plate and roll in each chicken wing.

Place on a baking sheet and bake for 30-35 minutes or until golden brown and cooked within.

Sprinkle with the cheese blend, green chilies, scallions, and jalapeño

pepper on top.

Serve immediately.

Nutrition Facts: Cal 802; Net Carbs 1.5g; Fat 59g; Protein 51g

Eggplant & Bacon Gratin

Ingredients for 4 servings

- 3 large eggplants, sliced
- 6 bacon slices, chopped
- ½ cup shredded Parmesan
- ½ cup crumbled feta cheese
- 1 tbsp dried oregano
- ¾ cup heavy cream
- 2 tbsp chopped parsley
- Salt and black pepper to taste

Instructions and Total Time: approx. 50 minutes

Preheat oven to 380 F.

Put bacon in a skillet and fry over medium heat until brown and crispy, 6 minutes.

Transfer to a plate.

Arrange half of eggplants in a greased baking sheet and season with

oregano, parsley, salt, and pepper.

Scatter half of bacon and half of feta cheese on top and repeat the layering

process using the remaining **Ingredients**.

In a bowl, combine heavy cream with half of the Parmesan cheese, and

spread on top of the layered **Ingredients**.

Sprinkle with the remaining Parmesan.

Bake until the cream is bubbly and the gratin golden, 20 minutes.

Serve.

Nutrition Facts: Cal 429; Net Carbs 1.7g; Fat 30g; Protein 16g

Bacon Wrapped Halloumi

Ingredients for 4 servings

- 16 bacon strips
- ½ lb halloumi cheese, cubed
- ½ cup swerve brown sugar
- ½ cup mayonnaise
- ¼ cup hot sauce

Instructions and Total Time: approx. 30 minutes

Place the bacon in a skillet and cook over medium heat on both sides until crisp, 5 minutes; transfer to a plate.

Wrap each halloumi cheese with a bacon strip and secure with a toothpick each.

Place on a baking sheet.

In a bowl, combine swerve brown sugar, mayonnaise, and hot sauce.

Pour the mixture all over the bacon-halloumi pieces and bake in the oven at
350 F for 10 minutes.
Serve chilled.
Nutrition Facts: Cal 351; Net Carbs 4.6g; Fat 24.9g; Protein 13g

Mini Sausages with Sweet Mustard Sauce

Ingredients for 4 servings

- 2 lb mini smoked sausages
- 3 tbsp almond flour
- 2 tsp mustard powder
- ¼ cup lemon juice
- ¼ cup white wine vinegar
- 1 cup swerve brown sugar
- 1 tsp tamari sauce

Instructions and Total Time: approx. 15 minutes

In a pot, combine swerve brown sugar, almond flour, and mustard.

Gradually stir in lemon juice, vinegar, and tamari sauce.

Bring to a boil over medium heat while stirring until thickened, 2 minutes.

Mix in sausages until properly coated.

Cook them for 5 minutes.

Serve warm.

Nutrition Facts: Cal 751; Net Carbs 7.2g; Fat 44.8g; Protein 24g

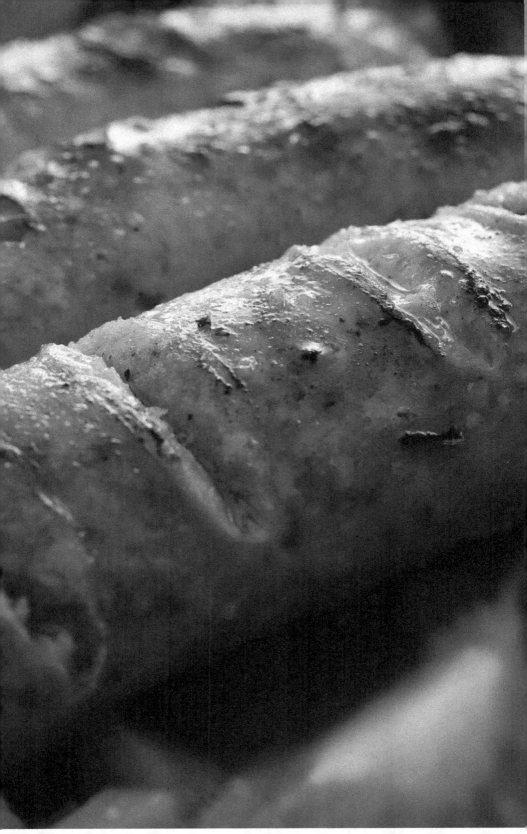

Pancetta & Broccoli Roast

Ingredients for 4 servings

- 6 pancetta slices, chopped
- 1 lb broccoli rabe, halved
- 2 tbsp olive oil
- ¼ tsp red chili flakes

Instructions and Total Time: approx. 40 minutes

Preheat oven to 420 F.

Place broccoli rabe in a greased baking sheet and top with pancetta.

Drizzle with olive oil, season to taste, and sprinkle with chili flakes.

Roast for 30 minutes.

Serve warm and enjoy!

Nutrition Facts: Cal 130; Net Carbs 0.2g; Fat 10g; Protein 6.8g

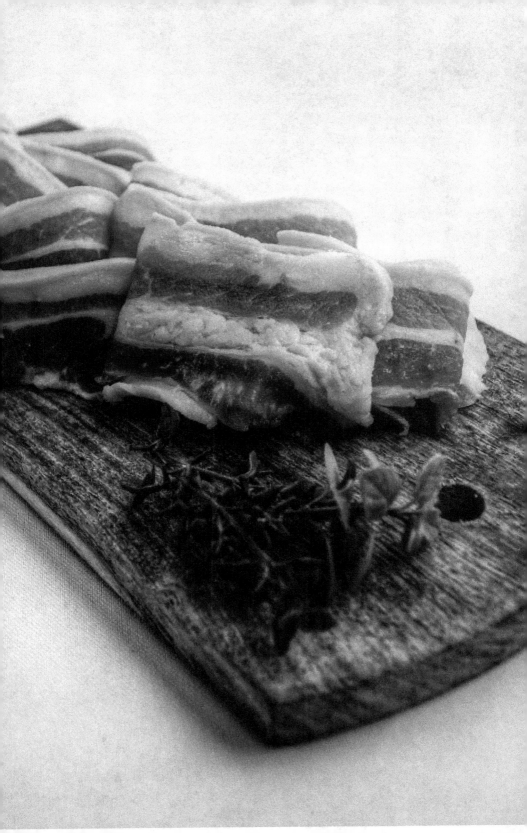

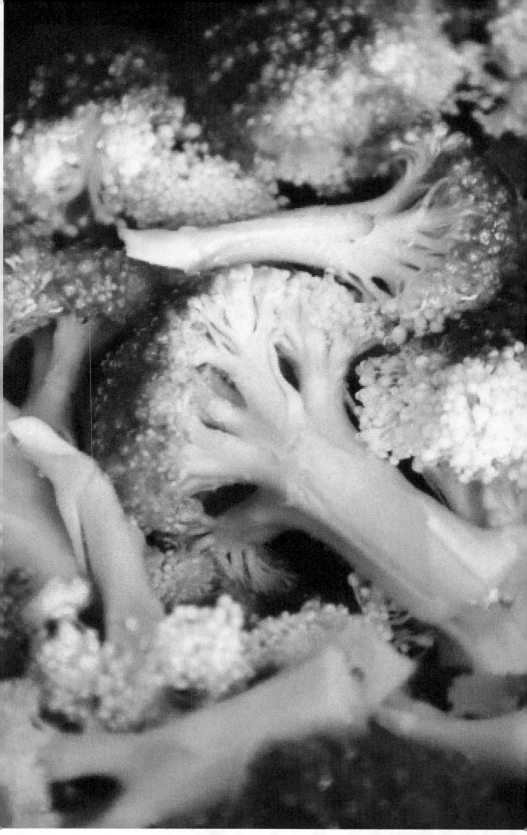

Mushroom & Kale Pierogis

Ingredients for 4 servings

- 2 oz fresh kale
- 3 oz bella mushrooms, sliced
- ½ cup cream cheese
- 2 cups Parmesan, grated
- 7 tbsp butter
- 2 garlic cloves, minced
- 1 small red onion, chopped
- 3 eggs
- ½ cup almond flour
- 4 tbsp coconut flour
- 1 tsp baking powder
- Salt and black pepper to taste

Instructions and Total Time: approx. 45 minutes

Melt 2 tbsp of butter in a skillet and sauté garlic, red onion, mushrooms, and kale for 5 minutes.

Season with salt and pepper and reduce the heat to low.

Stir in cream cheese and ½ cup of Parmesan cheese; simmer for 1 minute.

Set aside to cool.

In a bowl, combine almond and coconut flours, salt, and baking powder.

Put a pan over low heat and melt the remaining Parmesan cheese and butter.

Turn the heat off.

Pour the eggs in the cream mixture, continue stirring, while adding the flour mixture until a firm dough forms.

Mold the dough into balls, place on a chopping board, and use a rolling pin to flatten each into ½ inch thin round piece.

Spread a generous amount of stuffing on one-half of each dough, fold over the filling, and seal the dough with fingers. Brush with oil and bake for 20 minutes at 380 F.

Nutrition Facts: Cal 538; Net Carbs 6g; Fat 51g; Protein 18g

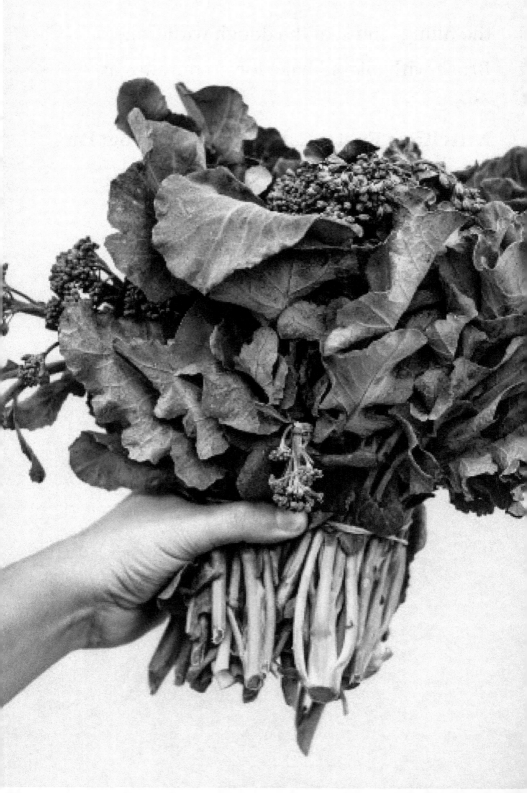

Chicken Ranch Pizza with Bacon & Basil

Ingredients for 4 servings

- 1 tbsp butter
- 2 chicken breasts
- 3 cups shredded mozzarella
- 3 tbsp cream cheese, softened
- ¾ cup almond flour
- 2 tbsp almond meal
- ¼ cup half and half
- 1 tbsp dry Ranch seasoning
- 3 bacon slices, chopped
- 6 fresh basil leaves

Instructions and Total Time: approx. 45 minutes

Preheat oven to 390 F.

Line a pizza pan with parchment paper.

Microwave 2 cups of mozzarella cheese and 2 tbsp of the cream cheese
for 30 seconds.

Mix in almond flour and almond meal.

Spread the "dough" on the pan and bake for 15 minutes.

In a bowl, mix butter, remaining cream cheese, half and half, and ranch
mix; set aside.

Heat a grill pan and cook the bacon for 5 minutes; set aside.

Grill the chicken in the pan on both sides for 10 minutes.

Remove to a plate, allow cooling and cut into thin slices.

Spread the ranch sauce on the pizza crust, followed by the chicken and
bacon, and then, the remaining mozzarella cheese and basil.

Bake for 5 minutes.

Serve sliced.

Nutrition Facts: Cal 531; Net Carbs 4g;

Fats 32g; Protein 62g

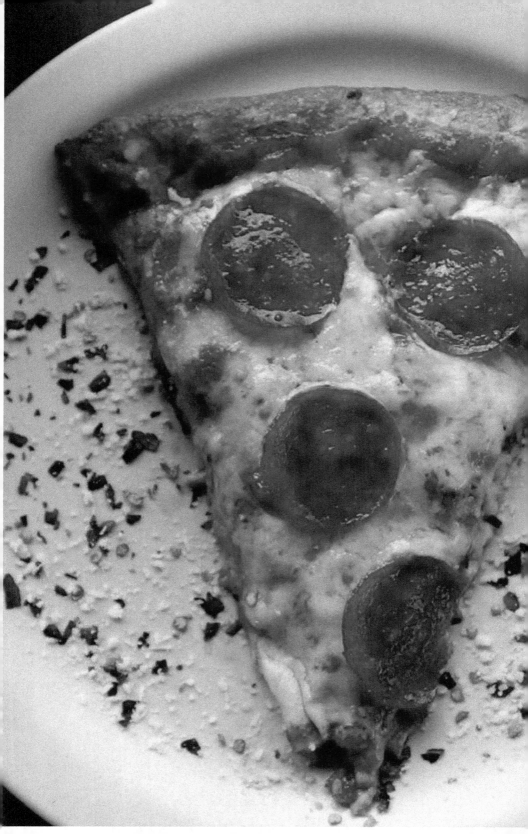

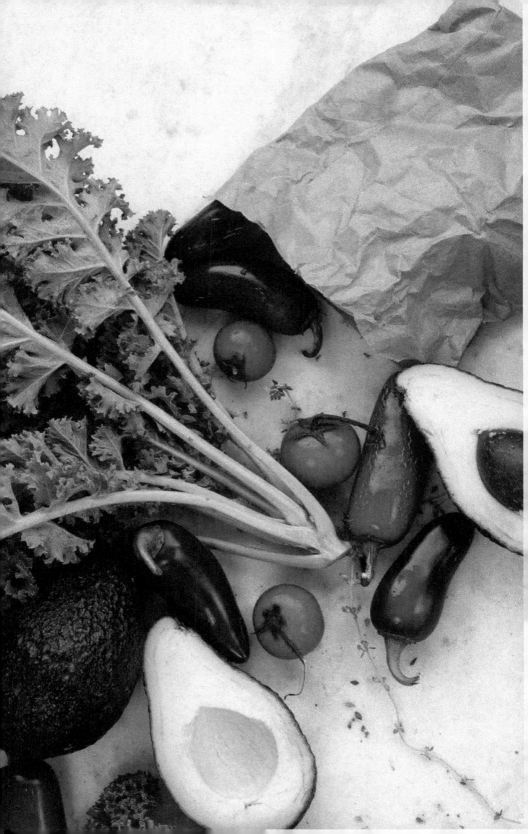

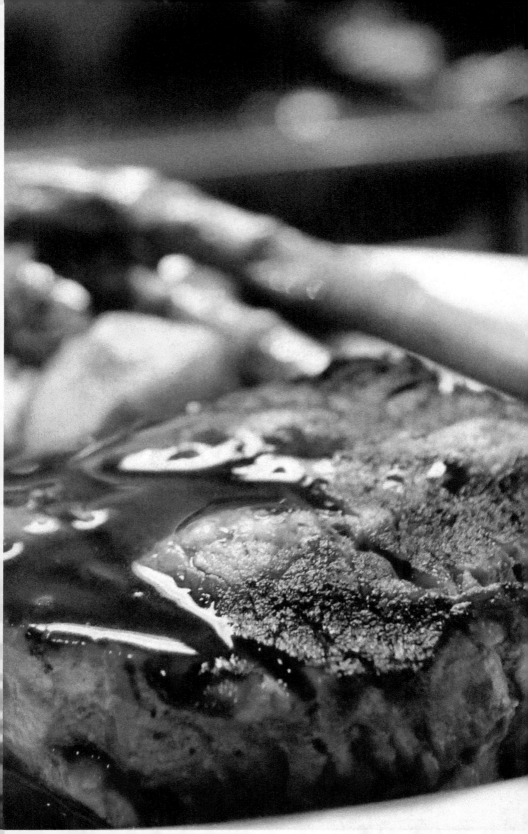

CPSIA information can be obtained
at www.ICGtesting.com
Printed in the USA
LVHW080528280521
688664LV00003B/312